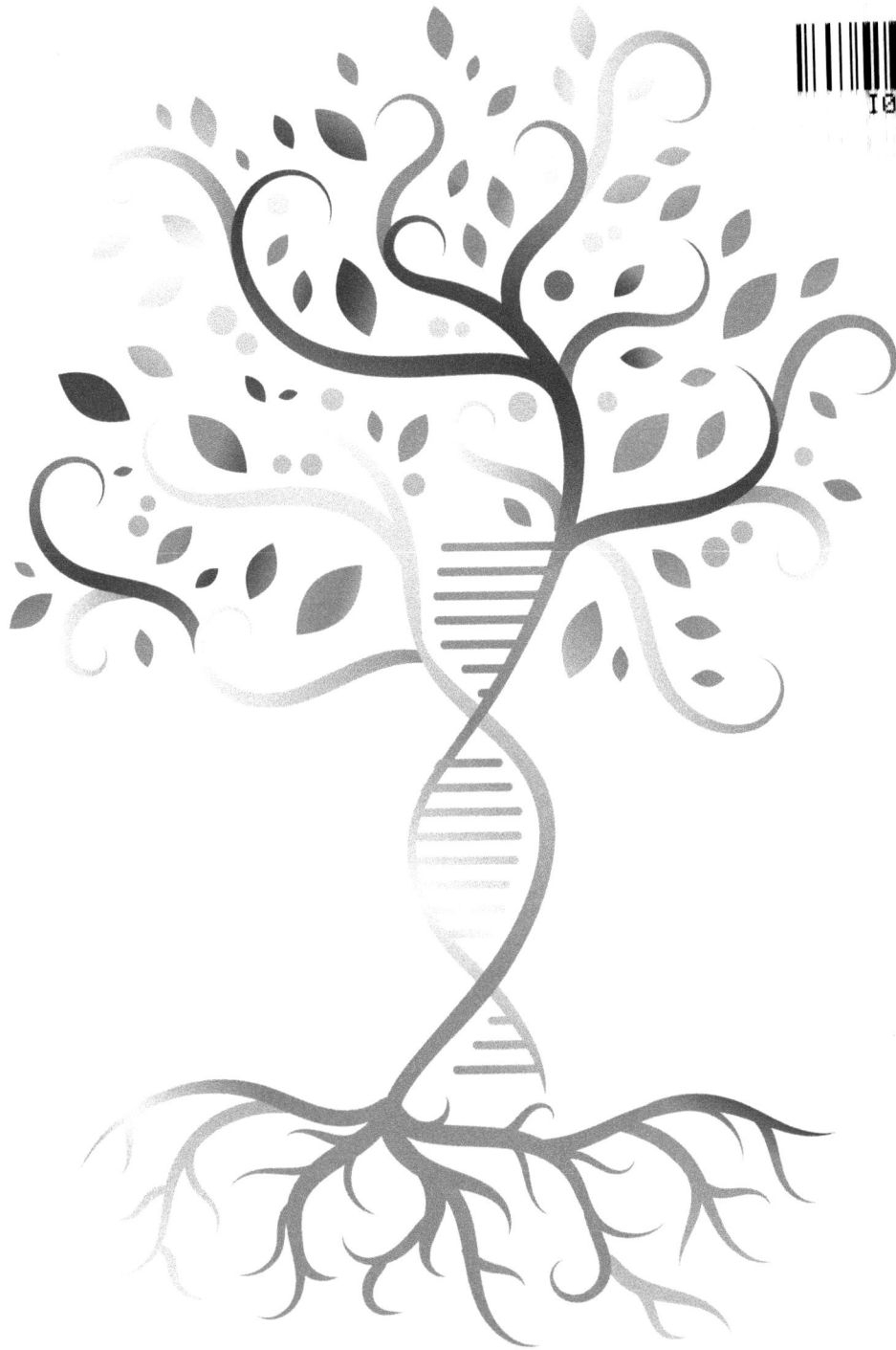

Personalized Medicine Care Planner
Creating Therapeutic Partnerships

Kara Ware

National Board, and Functional Medicine Certified Health Coach

This planner is designed to regain control of your health and well-being by assuming autonomy over implementing nutrition and lifestyle modifications, knowing your genetic vulnerabilities, timing medical interventions, understanding and budgeting medical costs, and driving health care decisions as an equal, therapeutic partner with your chosen provider(s). Use your planner to organize, track, and budget your personalized 90-day care plans.

info@braughlerbooks.com

First printing, 2023

ISBN: 978-1-955791-40-3

Ordering information: Special discounts are available on quantity purchases by bookstores, corporations, associations, and others. For details, contact the publisher at:

sales@braughlerbooks.com

or at 937-58-BOOKS

For questions or comments about this book, please write to:

info@braughlerbooks.com

To learn more about Kara Ware, visit karawarecoaching.com.

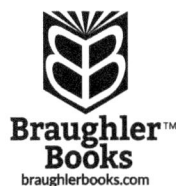

Braughler™
Books
braughlerbooks.com

Contents

Welcome to Personalized Medicine

Comprehensive and Coordinated Care Plans

Healthcare is fragmented! It is a terrifying maze to navigate. No medical provider or therapist can connect and layer all the pieces of a comprehensive care plan, implement, and sustain the plan for you. Regardless if you are the patient or a parent of a child living with a chronic condition/developmental delay, developing the skill set to design, document, track, and budget your comprehensive and coordinated care plan that fosters consistency and continuity of care is crucial. That is your responsibility, and it is challenging considering the abundance of information to sift and sort through and the number of professionals who are part of your care team. This care planner is your record-keeping journal, helping you track essential information about your dynamic personalized care plan. Use this planner to partner with family, educators, and medical providers on your personalized ninety-day care plans. You will find prompts to help you design, organize, document, track, and budget your personalized care plan. Use your planner to record your progress and successfully track where you have been so that you can make informed decisions about your next steps.

LIFESTYLE | GENETICS | MEDICAL

The interplay between your environment and your genetic code largely determines your health. Your environment includes your home atmosphere, stress, trauma, nutritional deficiencies, gut pathogens, and toxic exposures to mold, chemicals, and heavy metals in the food, air, water, personal care products, and everyday household items that interact with your genetic vulnerabilities and tip you into expressing symptoms of dis-ease. For personalized medicine to deliver on its promise of reversing once-thought dead-end diagnoses and placing symptoms of dis-ease into remission, lifestyle, genetics, and well-timed root cause medical interventions must be layered in an intelligent sequence.

Lifestyle

You have the most control over modifying your nutrition and environment. Placing priority on mastering the modifiable lifestyle changes in the following domains: nutrition, stress & resilience, sleep & relaxation, relationships & communication, time & money management, exercise & movement, as well as the mental, emotional, and spiritual facets of life, is the foundation to reclaiming your well-being and freedom. Placing priority on continuously peeling back lifestyle inflammation and creating an atmosphere conducive to healing drives the needle in optimizing outcomes. You will actually have to do fewer medical interventions if you take time before each medical protocol to peel back more environmental, emotional, nutritional, and lifestyle inflammation and strengthen everyone's physiological and psychological constitution.

Genetics

Nutrigenomics aims to guide more precise nutritional support by understanding your unique genetic code. SNPs (single nucleotide polymorphisms) or genetic variants are differences in a single DNA building block that makes each person unique. Like your eye and hair color physical traits, SNPs affect other traits like how well you metabolize or utilize, or transport essential key nutrients, metabolize caffeine or estrogen, detox toxic substrates, regulate the three metabolic hormones, your susceptibility to an overactive immune response, or your dopamine and serotonin bioavailability. It's important to know that SNPs or genetic variants are not good or bad; it depends on the environment that interacts with your genes. It's good news that you can modify your environment and modulate your gene expression! This is why modifying lifestyle factors, including the mental, emotional, and spiritual facets, is the foundation of good medicine. Genetic information deepens the personalization of your nutrition and lifestyle changes. You no longer have to guess what diet and lifestyle are proper for you. Genetics can help identify what essential nutrients you may have a higher demand for when stress, trauma, poor diet, toxicity, and other aggressive inflammatory triggers are present. Just because a vulnerability is in your genes (genetics) doesn't mean you have to express it (epigenetics).

Medical

Functional medicine's systems biology medical model offers strategy and advanced medical interventions and protocols to address vector-borne illnesses, detoxification of biotoxins, heavy metals, and chemicals, kill gut pathogens like viruses, bacteria, fungi, and parasites, induce cellular autophagy, and regenerate neuronal growth and synaptic connections. But before it's safe to implement another protocol to kill, detoxify, induce, and regenerate, it's intelligent to strengthen everyone's constitution (including parents) by peeling back more mental, emotional, spiritual, nutritional, and lifestyle inflammation. In addition, it's wise to get in the habit of keeping all of your chart summaries, lab results and receipts in a binder to keep track of your journey.

It is crucial you understand that no doctor or therapist can resolve your complaints. They are you guides. It is the responsibility of patients and parents to create comprehensive and coordinated care plans, which create consistency and continuity of care. When working with a medical provider, be sure to use your voice to co-create a reasonable treatment plan that matches your current emotional and financial ability.

Build Your Personalized Care Plan

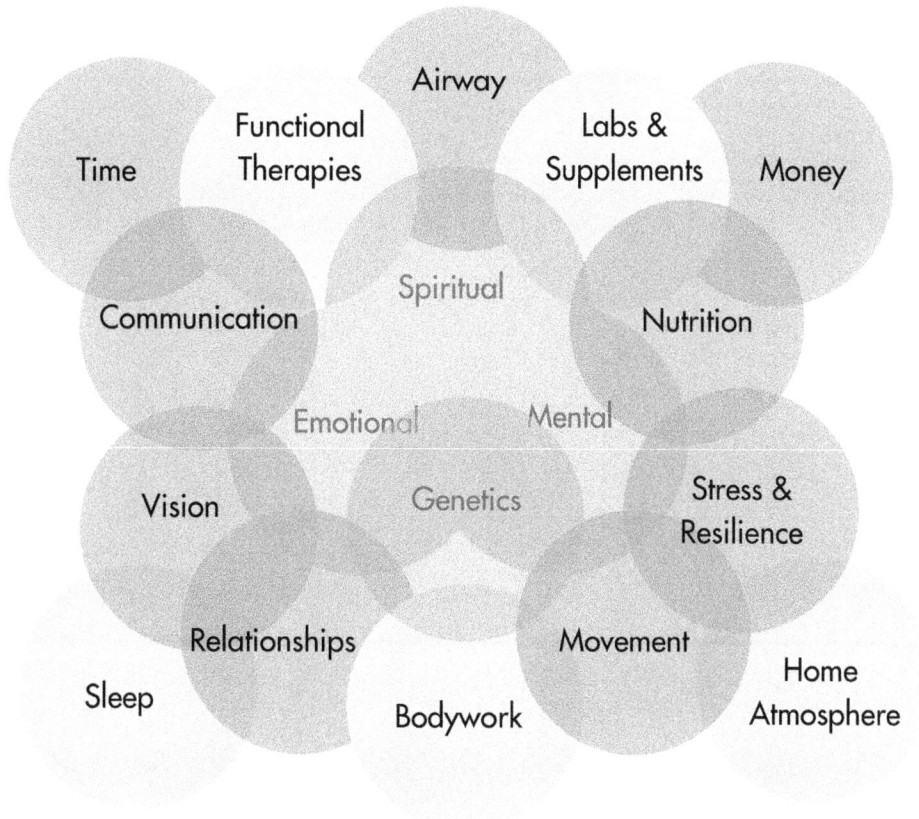

Airway

Functional Therapies

Labs & Supplements

Time

Money

Spiritual

Communication

Nutrition

Emotional

Mental

Vision

Genetics

Stress & Resilience

Relationships

Movement

Sleep

Bodywork

Home Atmosphere

Conventional medicine's approach to health care is disease-centric and is based on pharmaceuticals and/or procedures. Personalized medicine is person-centric and based on including the entire person, all biological and neurological systems, plus the mental, emotional, and spiritual facets. No one nutrition or lifestyle modification, supplement, or medical intervention in and of itself will resolve all your pains. It's an accumulation of all pieces to a comprehensive care plan, including the mental, emotional, and spiritual components, working in combination, allowing you to experience your desired results (gains).

Once you implement a nutrition or lifestyle change, maintain it just like completing a puzzle. Choose small steps, build momentum, feel good about what you are doing, rely on your strengths, seek support, and create consistency. Layering the right piece at the right time to work in combination with all the previous pieces is the right formula for healing. Choosing better feeling thoughts, to elevate your emotions, which improve your communication and direct your actions and habits, is the process of creating your desired destiny.

You can do this!

Current Ability
(motivation + competence + confidence)

ABILITY CREATES STABILITY

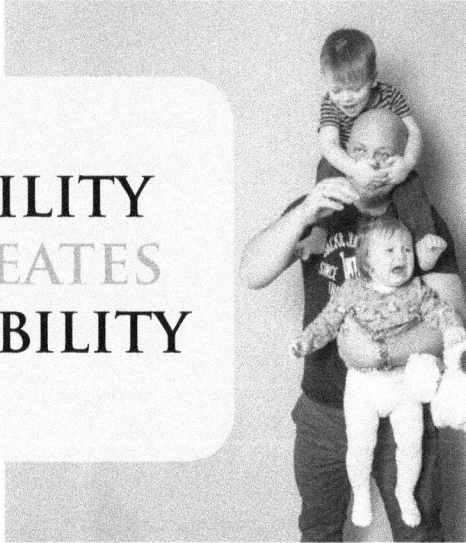

With so much information on gut health, the gut-brain axis, sources of inflammation, supplements, lab testing, and expensive therapies, it's common for patients and parents to feel overwhelmed. "What's right for me?" "Where do I start?" "I've been trying everything, and nothing is working." Overwhelm is a sign you are trying to make too many changes that do not match your current financial and emotional ability.

Get excited about mastering the basics. Choose pieces of a comprehensive care plan based on what you feel motivated to change, competent to change, and confident to change. Ask yourself, "What can I do?" "What is reasonable?" "What do I feel good about changing, implementing, and sustaining?" Over time, small steps add up to create positive change.

There is no quick fix when reversing debilitating chronic conditions and developmental delays. Get intentional by guiding your journey of hope and healing in an intelligent sequence to prepare your mind, body, spirit, and finances for more advanced medical interventions and therapies.

Creating a 3-month personalized and comprehensive care plan is the best way to become intentional. Creating a 90-day personalized care plan helps you complete what you set out to change. You can't do everything all at once, so choose what you can reasonably accomplish in 90-days. 90-days allow enough time to implement a few desired changes/interventions, become consistent, and stabilize your changes, so they integrate into your life and mindset. What once felt impossible will become reasonable. Stop grasping at straws! This is how you begin to find peace amid chaos. Every three months, evolve your personalized plan. Use this planner to organize, document, track, and budget your personalized 90-day plans based on your current ability.

"Healing isn't something you do, it's who you become." – Kara Ware

Write Your Key Concepts

Love
Freedom | Appreciation
Joy | Knowledge | Empowerment |
Passion
Enthusiasm | Eagerness | Happiness
Positive Expectations | Belief
Optimisim
Hopefulness
Contentment
Pessimism
Frustration | Impatience | Irritation
Overwhelm
Dissappointment
Worry
Anger
Blame
Revenge
Hatred | Rage
Jealousy
Insecurity | Guilt | Unworthiness
Fear | Grief | Depression | Despair | Powerlessness

Emotional Scale

Train Your Mind.
Reach for better feeling thoughts.

The Emotional Scale: An exercise to train your thoughts, and feelings to positively affect your words, actions, and habits.

A solution is not found by thinking and perseverating on the problem. The Hope for Healing workbook provides a self-directed neuroplasticity emotional scale exercise that guides you to find new ideas, thoughts, inspirations, and solutions to shape and steer your healing journey. This exercise helps you to lean into love, the greatest reason and motivator. It is a method to airlift you out of fear and allow love to be the underpinning to your decisions, words, actions, habits, character, and destiny. This is how you begin to affect your environment rather than reacting to the chaos and fear.

The more you practice reaching for better-feeling thoughts, the more your healing philosophy emerges. Your better-feeling thoughts become positive guiding thoughts and affirmations. We refer to these positive affirmations as key concepts; your philosophy of healing. Turn to your key concepts to catch yourself when you begin to downward spiral into fear-based emotions. Relying on your key concepts to interrupt and help you shift your emotional state is how you will create the internal and external healing atmosphere! What consumes your thoughts controls your life.

_____

_____

_____

_____

_____

_____

_____

_____

_____

_____

_____

Months 1-3

No one nutrition or lifestyle modification, supplement, or medical intervention in and of itself will resolve all your pains. It's an accumulation of all pieces to a comprehensive care plan, including the mental, emotional, and spiritual components, working together to create your desired results. So much positive change can happen in one year's time.

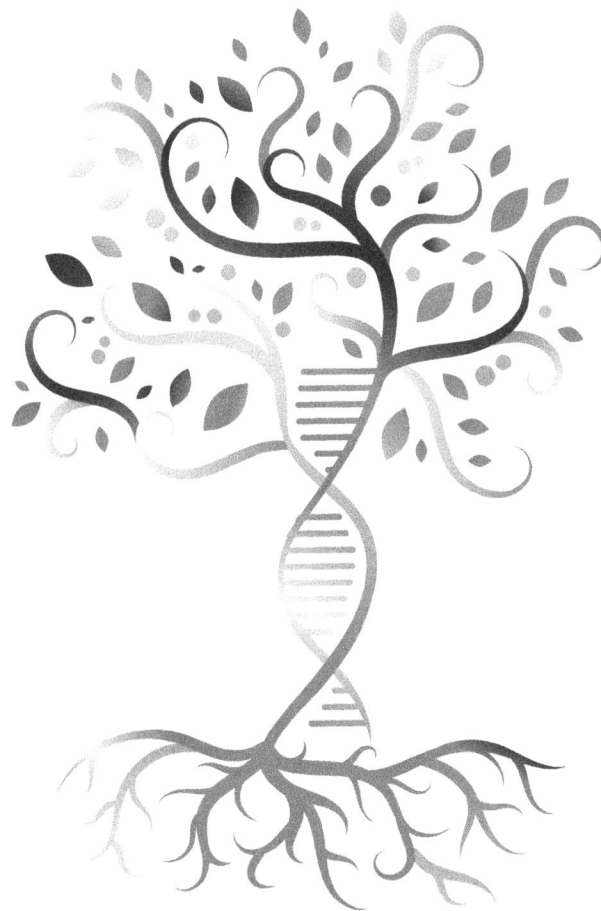

Modifiable Lifestyle Factors

What changes are you working on this month? Are the changes a match to your current ability? If you feel overwhelmed, remember to break down the changes into smaller, more achievable steps.

Month and Year: _____

SLEEP & RELAXATION

EXERCISE & MOVEMENT

STRESS & RESILIANCE

NUTRITION/LIFESTYLE

RELATIONSHIPS

Build Your 90-day Personalized Care Plan

Write your vision, goals, and motivators for your next 3-month care plan.

THERAPIES, BODYWORK, COUNSELING, ENERGY WORK, ETC

MENTAL | EMOTIONAL | SPIRITUAL

MEDICAL | GENETICS

Daily Supplements

Ask your provider in what order to start supplements. It's suggested to add one new supplement at a time. It is common to see an increase in symptoms. If it continues past 3-4 days, ask your doctor if you should reduce dosage/frequency, add in the next supplement to see if this balances the increase in symptoms or stop supplement.

Functions

- Binders for excreting toxins
- Drainage Support (liver, gallbladder, spleen, lungs)
- GI Support (digestion/absorption/biofilm/healing mucosal lining)
- Immune Support (Mast Cell Activation)
- Inflammation
- Lyme
- Metabolic and Insulin Homeostasis
- Methylation
- Microbial Load (fungi/bacteria/parasites/viral load)
- Neuroendocrine Support
- SNPs
- Vitamins & Minerals

Before Breakfast

Supplement	Dosage	Function	Price

Breakfast

Supplement	Dosage	Function	Price

Daily Supplements

Lunch

Supplement	Dosage	Function	Price

Dinner

Supplement	Dosage	Function	Price

Before Bed

Supplement	Dosage	Function	Price

			Total Price

Prescriptions and Compound Pharmacy

Drug-Nutrient Depletion: Did you know that common prescriptions have the potential to deplete critical nutrients? You can use this reference https://mytavin.com/ to learn more about the prescriptions you are currently taking and the possible drug-nutrient depletion. **Always** consult with your health care provider prior to making any changes to prescriptions or supplements.

Prescription	Dose	Reason	Side Effects	Drug-Nutrient Depletion	Cost

Questions to ask your health care provider:

PHARMACOGENOMICS

Pharmacogenomics: Adverse drug reactions are the 5th leading cause of death in the United States today. For over 20-years, the field of pharmacogenomics (PGx) has developed. PGx gives insight into how everyone's unique genetic profile effects how medication will work for them. Genetic factors account for up to 95% of an individual's drug response. Dr. Jamie Wilkey, PharmD says "When we don't look at how genetics play a role in medications for patients, then we are really just playing an intelligent guessing game to determine what medications are right for that individual. Often times, medications don't work or cause a lot of side effects because it's not the right prescription for the patients' genetic profile."

Care Plan Budget

Provider/Coaching Visits

1. _____ $ _____
2. _____ $ _____
3. _____ $ _____
4. _____ $ _____

Total: $ _____

Supplements & Compounded Rx ordered this month

1. _____ $ _____
2. _____ $ _____

Total: $ _____

Labs ordered this month

Document the Diagnostic Code for the ordered lab. Call the customer service number on your insurance card to make sure the diagnostic code is covered by your insurance. Most mental health diagnostic codes will not be covered by insurance. Be sure to ask your provider what code he/she has in your child's medical record. NOTE: Some lab work orders are known to NOT be covered by insurance, please ask your provider and prioritize labs so to fit within your monthly budget.

1. _____ Dx Code _____ $ _____
2. _____ Dx Code _____ $ _____
3. _____ Dx Code _____ $ _____

Total: $ _____

Counseling, Therapies and Bodywork

1. _____ $ _____
2. _____ $ _____
3. _____ $ _____
4. _____ $ _____

Total: $ _____

Total out-of-pocket medical expenses this month   Total: $ _____

Care Plan Notes

"The secret to change is to focus all of your energy, not on fighting the old, but on building the new." —SOCRATES

Care Plan Notes

"Parents are the ultimate role models for children. Every word, movement and action has an effect. No other person or outside force has a greater influence on a child than the parent." —Bob Keeshan

Month and Year:

Sunday	Monday	Tuesday	Wednesday

Personalized Medicine Care Planner

Thursday	Friday	Saturday

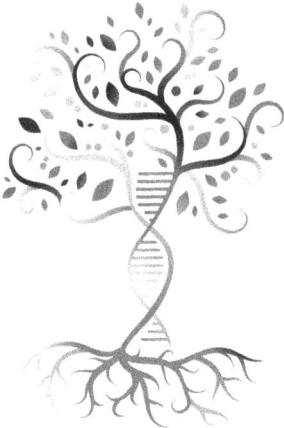

Remember to document when you start and stop supplements and record symptoms.

Remember to record regressions and positive gains!

List your current concerns:

_____

_____

_____

_____

_____

_____

_____

_____

_____

_____

_____

_____

_____

_____

Journal Entries

DATE:

DATE:

DATE:

Journal Entries

DATE:

DATE:

DATE:

DATE:

Month and Year:

Sunday	Monday	Tuesday	Wednesday

Thursday	Friday	Saturday

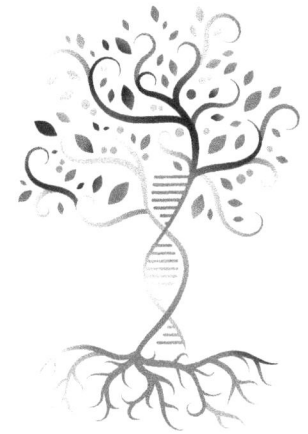

Remember to document when you start and stop supplements and record symptoms.

Remember to record regressions and positive gains!

List your current concerns:

_____

_____

_____

_____

_____

_____

_____

_____

_____

_____

_____

_____

_____

_____

_____

Journal Entries

DATE:

DATE:

DATE:

Journal Entries

Date:

Date:

Date:

Date:

Month and Year:

Sunday	Monday	Tuesday	Wednesday

Thursday	Friday	Saturday

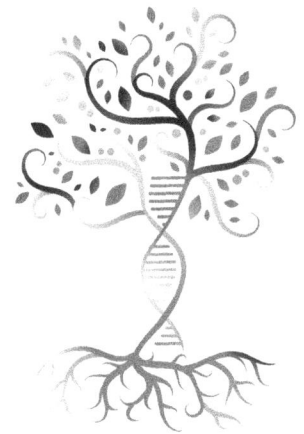

Remember to document when you start and stop supplements and record symptoms.

Remember to record regressions and positive gains!

List your current concerns:

_____

_____

_____

_____

_____

_____

_____

_____

_____

_____

_____

_____

_____

_____

_____

_____

Journal Entries

Date:

Date:

Date:

Journal Entries

DATE:

DATE:

DATE:

DATE:

Care Plan Update

Month: _____

CURRENT CONCERNS

MENTAL | EMOTIONAL | SPIRITUAL

MODIFIABLE LIFESTYLE FACTORS

GENETICS | MEDICAL | THERAPIES

SUPPLEMENT AND PRESCRIPTION QUESTIONS

STOOLS AND SLEEP

RECOGNIZABLE GAINS | IMPROVEMENTS

QUESTIONS FOR MY PROVIDER

90-days — Tell Your Story!

What's really changing the face of healthcare? The stories of profound healing from the patients and parents who have committed themselves to the personalized medicine's journey of healing and transformation. You have a story to tell. Write a chapter in your book.

Document Your Story

Months 4-6

Every three months, update your care plan by choosing the next nutrition and lifestyle changes that match your current motivation, competence, and confidence (current ability). Once you add a change to your plan, maintain it. This is called the Layering Method. The changes that may have initially felt impossible will soon enough become possible. It's highly recommended that you continuously become more devoted to mastering nutrition and lifestyle changes. As you continue your journey, you will layer more changes to work in combination with the previous three-month plan.

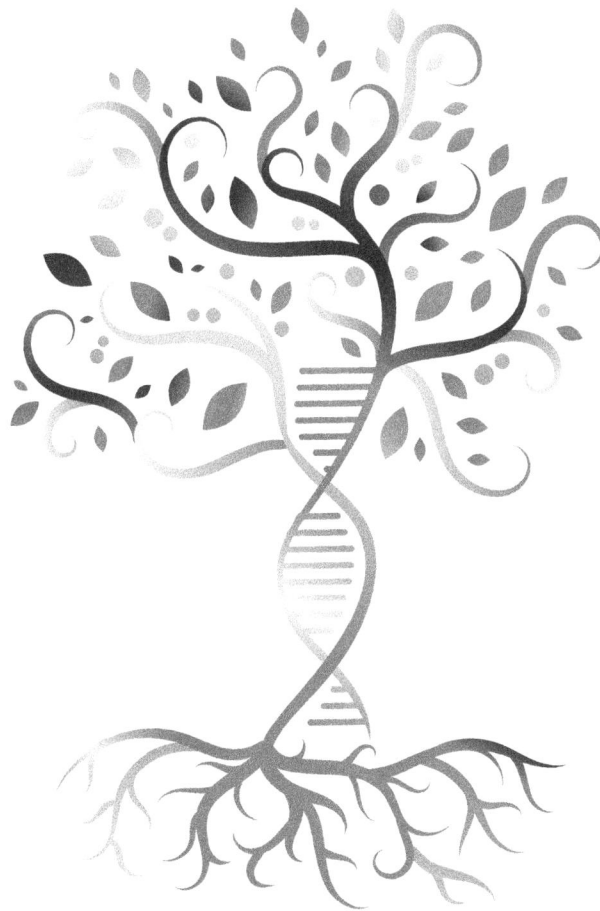

Modifiable Lifestyle Factors

What changes are you working on this month? Are the changes a match to your current ability? If you feel overwhelmed, remember to break down the changes into smaller, more achievable steps.

Month and Year: _____

SLEEP & RELAXATION

EXERCISE & MOVEMENT

STRESS & RESILIANCE

NUTRITION/LIFESTYLE

RELATIONSHIPS

Build Your 90-day Personalized Care Plan

Write your vision, goals, and motivators for your next 3-month care plan.

THERAPIES, BODYWORK, COUNSELING, ENERGY WORK, ETC

MENTAL | EMOTIONAL | SPIRITUAL

MEDICAL | GENETICS

Daily Supplements

Ask your provider in what order to start supplements. It's suggested to add one new supplement at a time. It is common to see an increase in symptoms. If it continues past 3-4 days, ask your doctor if you should reduce dosage/frequency, add in the next supplement to see if this balances the increase in symptoms or stop supplement.

Functions

- Binders for excreting toxins
- Drainage Support (liver, gallbladder, spleen, lungs)
- GI Support (digestion/absorption/biofilm/healing mucosal lining)
- Immune Support (Mast Cell Activation)
- Inflammation
- Lyme
- Metabolic and Insulin Homeostasis
- Methylation
- Microbial Load (fungi/bacteria/parasites/viral load)
- Neuroendocrine Support
- SNPs
- Vitamins & Minerals

	Supplement	Dosage	Function	Price
Before Breakgfast				

	Supplement	Dosage	Function	Price
Breakfast				

Daily Supplements

Lunch	Supplement	Dosage	Function	Price

Dinner	Supplement	Dosage	Function	Price

Before Bed	Supplement	Dosage	Function	Price

	Total Price

Prescriptions and Compound Pharmacy

Drug-Nutrient Depletion: Did you know that common prescriptions have the potential to deplete critical nutrients? You can use this reference https://mytavin.com/ to learn more about the prescriptions you are currently taking and the possible drug-nutrient depletion. **Always** consult with your health care provider prior to making any changes to prescriptions or supplements.

Prescription	Dose	Reason	Side Effects	Drug-Nutrient Depletion	Cost

Questions to ask your health care provider:

PHARMACOGENOMICS

Pharmacogenomics: Adverse drug reactions are the 5th leading cause of death in the United States today. For over 20-years, the field of pharmacogenomics (PGx) has developed. PGx gives insight into how everyone's unique genetic profile effects how medication will work for them. Genetic factors account for up to 95% of an individual's drug response. Dr. Jamie Wilkey, PharmD says "When we don't look at how genetics play a role in medications for patients, then we are really just playing an intelligent guessing game to determine what medications are right for that individual. Often times, medications don't work or cause a lot of side effects because it's not the right prescription for the patients' genetic profile."

Care Plan Budget

Provider/Coaching Visits

1. _____ $ _____
2. _____ $ _____
3. _____ $ _____
4. _____ $ _____

Total: $ _____

Supplements & Compounded Rx ordered this month

1. _____ $ _____
2. _____ $ _____

Total: $ _____

Labs ordered this month

Document the Diagnostic Code for the ordered lab. Call the customer service number on your insurance card to make sure the diagnostic code is covered by your insurance. Most mental health diagnostic codes will not be covered by insurance. Be sure to ask your provider what code he/she has in your child's medical record. NOTE: Some lab work orders are known to NOT be covered by insurance, please ask your provider and prioritize labs so to fit within your monthly budget.

1. _____ Dx Code _____ $ _____
2. _____ Dx Code _____ $ _____
3. _____ Dx Code _____ $ _____

Total: $ _____

Counseling, Therapies and Bodywork

1. _____ $ _____
2. _____ $ _____
3. _____ $ _____
4. _____ $ _____

Total: $ _____

Total out-of-pocket medical expenses this month   Total: $ _____

Care Plan Notes

"If you focus on results, you will never change. If you focus on change, you will get results." —Bob Dixon

Care Plan Notes

"The significant problems of our time won't be solved at the same level of thinking that created them." —ALBERT EINSTEIN

Month and Year: _____

Sunday	Monday	Tuesday	Wednesday

Personalized Medicine Care Planner

Thursday	Friday	Saturday

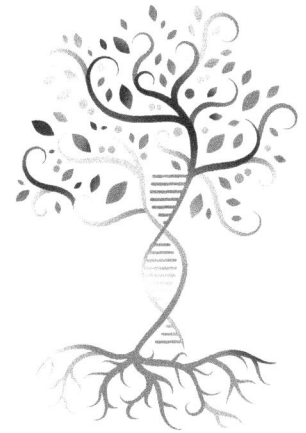

Remember to document when you start and stop supplements and record symptoms.

Remember to record regressions and positive gains!

List your current concerns:

_____

_____

_____

_____

_____

_____

_____

_____

_____

_____

_____

_____

_____

_____

_____

_____

_____

Journal Entries

DATE:

DATE:

DATE:

Journal Entries

Date:

Date:

Date:

Date:

Month and Year:

Sunday	Monday	Tuesday	Wednesday

Thursday	Friday	Saturday

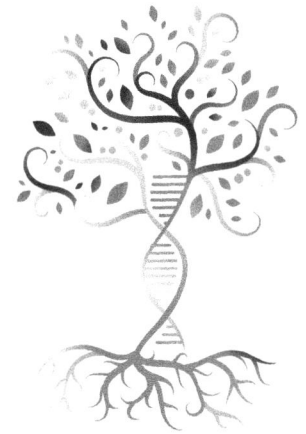

Remember to document when you start and stop supplements and record symptoms.

Remember to record regressions and positive gains!

List your current concerns:

_____

_____

_____

_____

_____

_____

_____

_____

_____

_____

_____

_____

_____

_____

_____

Journal Entries

DATE:

DATE:

DATE:

Journal Entries

DATE:

DATE:

DATE:

DATE:

Month and Year: _____

Sunday	Monday	Tuesday	Wednesday

Personalized Medicine Care Planner

Thursday	Friday	Saturday

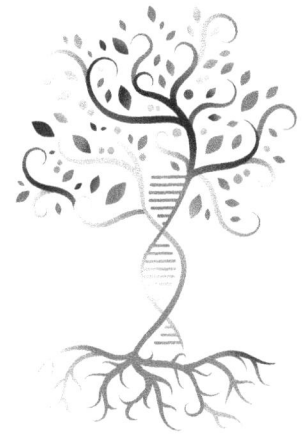

Remember to document when you start and stop supplements and record symptoms.

Remember to record regressions and positive gains!

List your current concerns:

_____

_____

_____

_____

_____

_____

_____

_____

_____

_____

_____

_____

_____

_____

_____

_____

Journal Entries

DATE:

DATE:

DATE:

Journal Entries

DATE:

DATE:

DATE:

DATE:

Care Plan Update

CURRENT CONCERNS

MENTAL | EMOTIONAL | SPIRITUAL

MODIFIABLE LIFESTYLE FACTORS

GENETICS | MEDICAL | THERAPIES

SUPPLEMENT AND PRESCRIPTION QUESTIONS

STOOLS AND SLEEP

RECOGNIZABLE GAINS | IMPROVEMENTS

QUESTIONS FOR MY PROVIDER

90-days — Tell Your Story!

What's really changing the face of healthcare? The stories of profound healing from the patients and parents who have committed themselves to the personalized medicine's journey of healing and transformation. You have a story to tell. Write a chapter in your book.

Document Your Story

Section Three
Months 7-9

The secret to success is building momentum by making small changes that feel easy and within your current emotional and financial ability, sustaining those changes, and repeating the process. These small changes add up to making big changes.

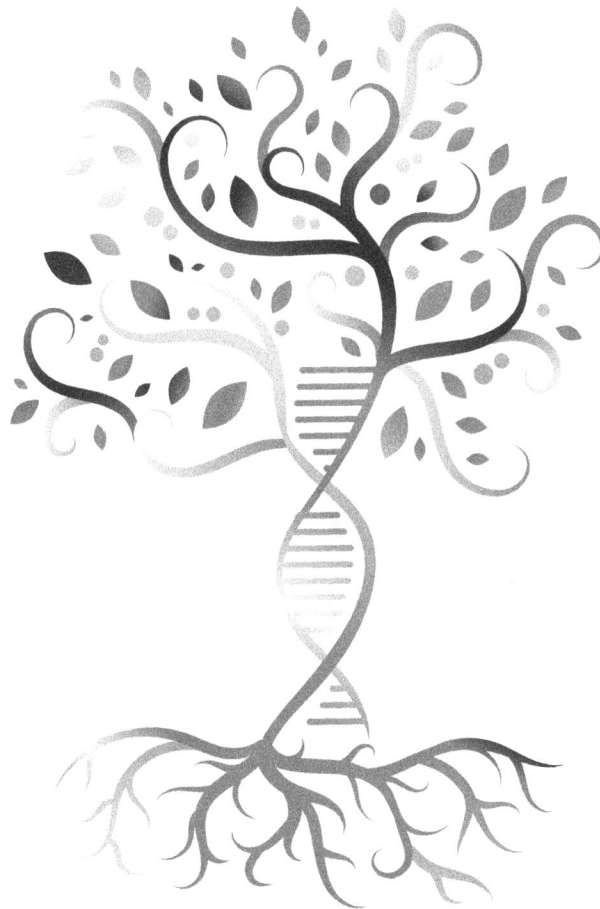

Modifiable Lifestyle Factors

What changes are you working on this month? Are the changes a match to your current ability? If you feel overwhelmed, remember to break down the changes into smaller, more achievable steps.

Month and Year: _____

SLEEP & RELAXATION

EXERCISE & MOVEMENT

STRESS & RESILIANCE

NUTRITION/LIFESTYLE

RELATIONSHIPS

Build Your 90-day Personalized Care Plan

Write your vision, goals, and motivators for your next 3-month care plan.

THERAPIES, BODYWORK, COUNSELING, ENERGY WORK, ETC

MENTAL | EMOTIONAL | SPIRITUAL

MEDICAL | GENETICS

Daily Supplements

Ask your provider in what order to start supplements. It's suggested to add one new supplement at a time. It is common to see an increase in symptoms. If it continues past 3-4 days, ask your doctor if you should reduce dosage/frequency, add in the next supplement to see if this balances the increase in symptoms or stop supplement.

Functions

- Binders for excreting toxins
- Drainage Support (liver, gallbladder, spleen, lungs)
- GI Support (digestion/absorption/biofilm/healing mucosal lining)
- Immune Support (Mast Cell Activation)
- Inflammation
- Lyme
- Metabolic and Insulin Homeostasis
- Methylation
- Microbial Load (fungi/bacteria/parasites/viral load)
- Neuroendocrine Support
- SNPs
- Vitamins & Minerals

Before Breakgfast

Supplement	Dosage	Function	Price

Breakfast

Supplement	Dosage	Function	Price

Daily Supplements

Lunch	Supplement	Dosage	Function	Price

Dinner	Supplement	Dosage	Function	Price

Before Bed	Supplement	Dosage	Function	Price

	Total Price

Prescriptions and Compound Pharmacy

Drug-Nutrient Depletion: Did you know that common prescriptions have the potential to deplete critical nutrients? You can use this reference https://mytavin.com/ to learn more about the prescriptions you are currently taking and the possible drug-nutrient depletion. **Always** consult with your health care provider prior to making any changes to prescriptions or supplements.

Prescription	Dose	Reason	Side Effects	Drug-Nutrient Depletion	Cost

Questions to ask your health care provider:

PHARMACOGENOMICS

Pharmacogenomics: Adverse drug reactions are the 5th leading cause of death in the United States today. For over 20-years, the field of pharmacogenomics (PGx) has developed. PGx gives insight into how everyone's unique genetic profile effects how medication will work for them. Genetic factors account for up to 95% of an individual's drug response. Dr. Jamie Wilkey, PharmD says "When we don't look at how genetics play a role in medications for patients, then we are really just playing an intelligent guessing game to determine what medications are right for that individual. Often times, medications don't work or cause a lot of side effects because it's not the right prescription for the patients' genetic profile."

Care Plan Budget

Provider/Coaching Visits

1. _____ $ _____

2. _____ $ _____

3. _____ $ _____

4. _____ $ _____

Total: $ _____

Supplements & Compounded Rx ordered this month

1. _____ $ _____

2. _____ $ _____

Total: $ _____

Labs ordered this month

Document the Diagnostic Code for the ordered lab. Call the customer service number on your insurance card to make sure the diagnostic code is covered by your insurance. Most mental health diagnostic codes will not be covered by insurance. Be sure to ask your provider what code he/she has in your child's medical record. NOTE: Some lab work orders are known to NOT be covered by insurance, please ask your provider and prioritize labs so to fit within your monthly budget.

1. _____ Dx Code _____ $ _____

2. _____ Dx Code _____ $ _____

3. _____ Dx Code _____ $ _____

Total: $ _____

Counseling, Therapies and Bodywork

1. _____ $ _____

2. _____ $ _____

3. _____ $ _____

4. _____ $ _____

Total: $ _____

Total out-of-pocket medical expenses this month Total: $ _____

Care Plan Notes

"Old ways won't open new doors." —UNKNOWN

Care Plan Notes

"Simplicity will convert the initial boost of enthusiasm into endurance for the long journey." —Kara Ware

Month and Year:

Sunday	Monday	Tuesday	Wednesday

Thursday	Friday	Saturday

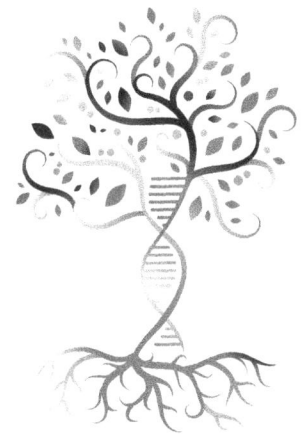

Remember to document when you start and stop supplements and record symptoms.

Remember to record regressions and positive gains!

List your current concerns:

_____

_____

_____

_____

_____

_____

_____

_____

_____

_____

_____

_____

_____

_____

_____

_____

_____

_____

Journal Entries

DATE:

DATE:

DATE:

Journal Entries

DATE:

DATE:

DATE:

DATE:

Sunday	Monday	Tuesday	Wednesday

Personalized Medicine Care Planner

Thursday	Friday	Saturday

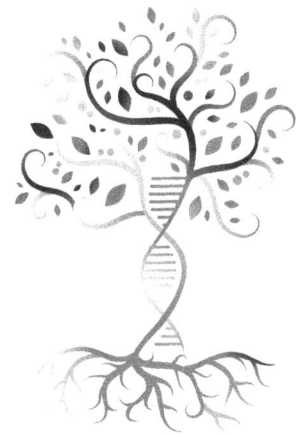

Remember to document when you start and stop supplements and record symptoms.

Remember to record regressions and positive gains!

List your current concerns:

_____

_____

_____

_____

_____

_____

_____

_____

_____

_____

_____

_____

_____

_____

_____

Journal Entries

DATE:

DATE:

DATE:

Journal Entries

DATE:

DATE:

DATE:

DATE:

Month and Year:

Sunday	Monday	Tuesday	Wednesday

Thursday	Friday	Saturday

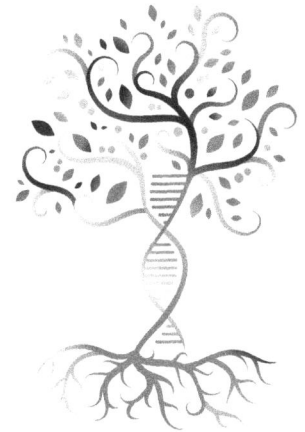

Remember to document when you start and stop supplements and record symptoms.

Remember to record regressions and positive gains!

List your current concerns:

_____

_____

_____

_____

_____

_____

_____

_____

_____

_____

_____

_____

_____

_____

_____

_____

Journal Entries

DATE:

DATE:

DATE:

Journal Entries

DATE:

DATE:

DATE:

DATE:

Care Plan Update

Month: _____

CURRENT CONCERNS

MENTAL | EMOTIONAL | SPIRITUAL

MODIFIABLE LIFESTYLE FACTORS

GENETICS | MEDICAL | THERAPIES

SUPPLEMENT AND PRESCRIPTION QUESTIONS

STOOLS AND SLEEP

RECOGNIZABLE GAINS | IMPROVEMENTS

QUESTIONS FOR MY PROVIDER

90-days — Tell Your Story!

What's really changing the face of healthcare? The stories of profound healing from the patients and parents who have committed themselves to the personalized medicine's journey of healing and transformation. You have a story to tell. Write a chapter in your book.

Document Your Story

Section Four
Months 10-12

Your healthcare is not an expense, it is an investment. Remember to prioritize the person you are becoming rather than your end-desired outcome. Use your key concepts to transform your greatest challenge into your greatest teacher to become the best, most courageous version of yourself!

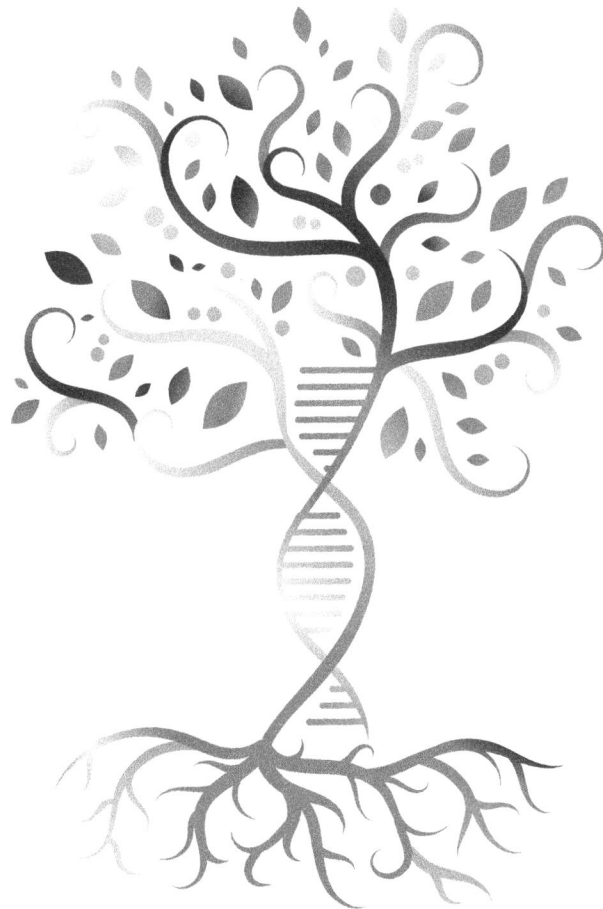

Modifiable Lifestyle Factors

What changes are you working on this month? Are the changes a match to your current ability? If you feel overwhelmed, remember to break down the changes into smaller, more achievable steps.

Month and Year: _____

SLEEP & RELAXATION

EXERCISE & MOVEMENT

STRESS & RESILIANCE

NUTRITION/LIFESTYLE

RELATIONSHIPS

Build Your 90-day Personalized Care Plan

Write your vision, goals, and motivators for your next 3-month care plan.

THERAPIES, BODYWORK, COUNSELING, ENERGY WORK, ETC

MENTAL | EMOTIONAL | SPIRITUAL

MEDICAL | GENETICS

Daily Supplements

Ask your provider in what order to start supplements. It's suggested to add one new supplement at a time. It is common to see an increase in symptoms. If it continues past 3-4 days, ask your doctor if you should reduce dosage/frequency, add in the next supplement to see if this balances the increase in symptoms or stop supplement.

Functions

- Binders for excreting toxins
- Drainage Support (liver, gallbladder, spleen, lungs)
- GI Support (digestion/absorption/biofilm/healing mucosal lining)
- Immune Support (Mast Cell Activation)
- Inflammation
- Lyme

- Metabolic and Insulin Homeostasis
- Methylation
- Microbial Load (fungi/bacteria/parasites/viral load)
- Neuroendocrine Support
- SNPs
- Vitamins & Minerals

Before Breakfast

Supplement	Dosage	Function	Price

Breakfast

Supplement	Dosage	Function	Price

Daily Supplements

Lunch

Supplement	Dosage	Function	Price

Dinner

Supplement	Dosage	Function	Price

Before Bed

Supplement	Dosage	Function	Price

			Total Price

Prescriptions and Compound Pharmacy

Drug-Nutrient Depletion: Did you know that common prescriptions have the potential to deplete critical nutrients? You can use this reference https://mytavin.com/ to learn more about the prescriptions you are currently taking and the possible drug-nutrient depletion. **Always** consult with your health care provider prior to making any changes to prescriptions or supplements.

Prescription	Dose	Reason	Side Effects	Drug-Nutrient Depletion	Cost

Questions to ask your
health care provider:

PHARMACOGENOMICS

Pharmacogenomics: Adverse drug reactions are the 5th leading cause of death in the United States today. For over 20-years, the field of pharmacogenomics (PGx) has developed. PGx gives insight into how everyone's unique genetic profile effects how medication will work for them. Genetic factors account for up to 95% of an individual's drug response. Dr. Jamie Wilkey, PharmD says "When we don't look at how genetics play a role in medications for patients, then we are really just playing an intelligent guessing game to determine what medications are right for that individual. Often times, medications don't work or cause a lot of side effects because it's not the right prescription for the patients' genetic profile."

Care Plan Budget

Provider/Coaching Visits

1. _____ $ _____

2. _____ $ _____

3. _____ $ _____

4. _____ $ _____

Total: $ _____

Supplements & Compounded Rx ordered this month

1. _____ $ _____

2. _____ $ _____

Total: $ _____

Labs ordered this month

Document the Diagnostic Code for the ordered lab. Call the customer service number on your insurance card to make sure the diagnostic code is covered by your insurance. Most mental health diagnostic codes will not be covered by insurance. Be sure to ask your provider what code he/she has in your child's medical record. NOTE: Some lab work orders are known to NOT be covered by insurance, please ask your provider and prioritize labs so to fit within your monthly budget.

1. _____ Dx Code _____ $ _____

2. _____ Dx Code _____ $ _____

3. _____ Dx Code _____ $ _____

Total: $ _____

Counseling, Therapies and Bodywork

1. _____ $ _____

2. _____ $ _____

3. _____ $ _____

4. _____ $ _____

Total: $ _____

Total out-of-pocket medical expenses this month   Total: $ _____

Care Plan Notes

"All truth passes through three stages. First, it is ridiculed. Second, it is violently opposed. Third, it is accepted as being self-evident." —ARTHUR SCHOPENHAUER

Care Plan Notes

"Whether you think you can or that you can't, you are usually right."
—HENRY FORD

Month and Year: _____

Sunday	Monday	Tuesday	Wednesday

Thursday	Friday	Saturday

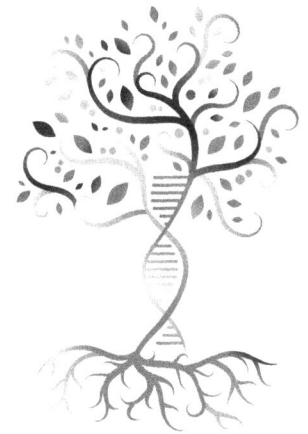

Remember to document when you start and stop supplements and record symptoms.

Remember to record regressions and positive gains!

List your current concerns:

_____

_____

_____

_____

_____

_____

_____

_____

_____

_____

_____

_____

_____

_____

_____

_____

Journal Entries

DATE:

DATE:

DATE:

Journal Entries

DATE:

DATE:

DATE:

DATE:

Month and Year: _____

Sunday	Monday	Tuesday	Wednesday

Thursday	Friday	Saturday

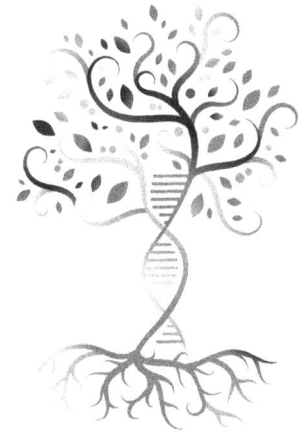

Remember to document when you start and stop supplements and record symptoms.

Remember to record regressions and positive gains!

List your current concerns:

_____
_____
_____
_____

_____
_____
_____
_____
_____
_____
_____
_____
_____
_____
_____

Journal Entries

DATE:

DATE:

DATE:

Journal Entries

Date:

Date:

Date:

Date:

Month and Year: _____

Sunday	Monday	Tuesday	Wednesday

Thursday	Friday	Saturday

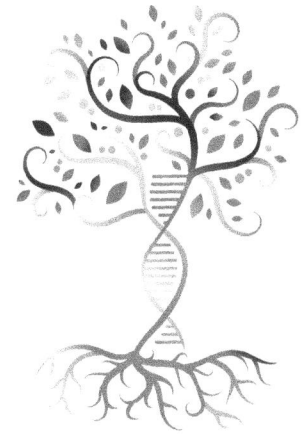

Remember to document when you start and stop supplements and record symptoms.

Remember to record regressions and positive gains!

List your current concerns:

_____

_____

_____

_____

_____

_____

_____

_____

_____

_____

_____

_____

_____

_____

_____

Journal Entries

DATE:

DATE:

DATE:

Journal Entries

DATE:

DATE:

DATE:

DATE:

Care Plan Update

Month: _____

CURRENT CONCERNS

MENTAL | EMOTIONAL | SPIRITUAL

MODIFIABLE LIFESTYLE FACTORS

GENETICS | MEDICAL | THERAPIES

SUPPLEMENT AND PRESCRIPTION QUESTIONS

STOOLS AND SLEEP

RECOGNIZABLE GAINS | IMPROVEMENTS

QUESTIONS FOR MY PROVIDER

90-days — Tell Your Story!

What's really changing the face of healthcare? The stories of profound healing from the patients and parents who have committed themselves to the personalized medicine's journey of healing and transformation. You have a story to tell. Write a chapter in your book.

Document Your Story

About the Author

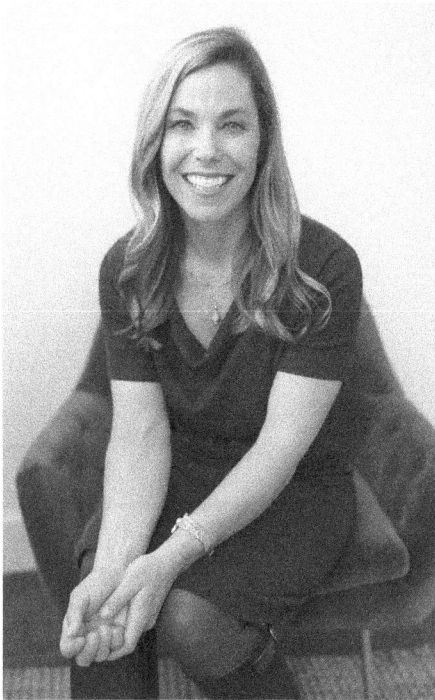

Kara Ware, a National Board and Functional Medicine Health Coach, has spent nearly two decades healing her son of the underlying causes creating the symptoms commonly referred to as Autism.

She did not accept the limiting belief there was nothing she could do for her son. Her son looked like he was in unbearable pain. She knew there must be something she could do to help him feel better, and therefore, behave better.

In times of dial-up internet and flip phones that did not text, let alone take photos and videos, she was divinely guided to learn about the sources of inflammation that were causing his pain and intolerable and terrifying Autistic behaviors and symptoms and how to intelligently and safely layer interventions to work in combination.

Kara discovered there were even more underlying conditions than Leaky Gut, Vitamin and Mineral Depletion, Microbial Overload, Suppressed Immune System, Heavy Metal and Mold Toxicity, Lyme Disease, etc.

She found her thoughts, which created her words, and then her actions which created her habits, which then created an atmosphere of healing was what ultimately allowed Kara to accomplish what many say is impossible.

When her perspective changed, and her anger turned to embracing what this journey had come to teach, the healing began. She learned her son came to teach her this shift from fear to love and how to support her family to thrive in today's environment.

This workbook is the accumulation of what Kara found and was willing to do to heal her son from this once thought dead-end diagnosis. Many pieces may seem insignificant; however, when all the nutrition and lifestyle and genetics and medical changes are layered in overtime to work in combination, and when love is the motivator, and the home becomes the headquarters for healing, miracles will happen.

* 9 7 8 1 9 5 5 7 9 1 4 0 3 *